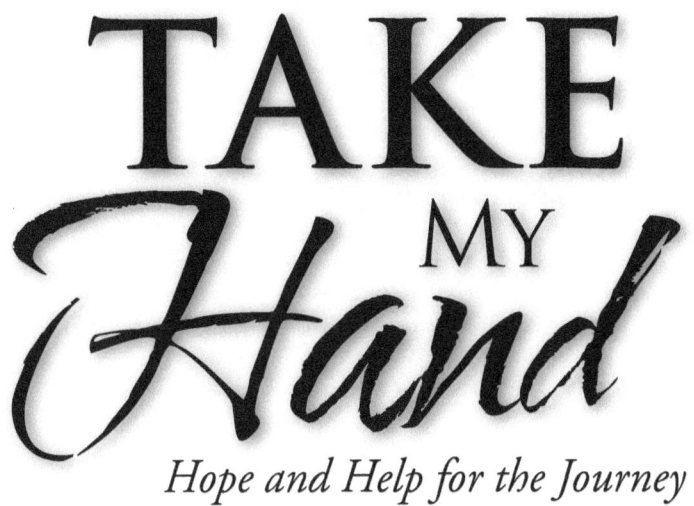

# TAKE MY Hand

*Hope and Help for the Journey*

## BETH WILSON

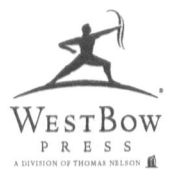

WESTBOW
PRESS
A DIVISION OF THOMAS NELSON

Scriptures taken from the Holy Bible, New International Version®, NIV®. Copyright © 1973, 1978, 1984, 2011 by Biblica, Inc.™ Used by permission of Zondervan. All rights reserved worldwide. www.zondervan.com The "NIV" and "New International Version" are trademarks registered in the United States Patent and Trademark Office by Biblica, Inc.™

WestBow Press books may be ordered through booksellers or by contacting:

WestBow Press
A Division of Thomas Nelson
1663 Liberty Drive
Bloomington, IN 47403
www.westbowpress.com
1-(866) 928-1240

ISBN: 978-1-4497-9348-7 (sc)
ISBN: 978-1-4497-9347-0 (e)

Library of Congress Control Number: 2013907669

Printed in the United States of America.

WestBow Press rev. date: 04/30/2013

To Florene Tomei—you fought the good fight,
you stayed true to the end, and you received the prize.

# Preface

*Dear Friend,*

*As I was getting ready to go to church, I had an incredible overwhelming feeling to write about my breast cancer experience. I laughed about the absurd idea because I can't put two sentences together that make sense. I called my friend Sherry who is an absolute wordsmith and she said I should do it.*

*I thought "Just another hair brain idea that will go nowhere." It is easy to talk about projects but it takes work to complete them.*

*So I get into my car and I am driving to church and I have to pull over and find a pen and paper because I was compelled to write some things down. And it has been that way through the entire book. I have put it aside and then had to, had to pick it back up again. A friend said "Even if I never publish, it will be good therapy for me." I scoffed at the idea. I didn't want therapy and I didn't want to write a book.*

*Well, here it is. It demanded to be written. I don't understand why but I do believe God has a purpose. Truly the only thing I felt I had to offer was complete openness. I want this to reflect exactly how I felt, what I thought, and how I reconciled the two. I tried to be honest even when it was ugly.*

*I have written to you so you could know the truth and not feel alone in your journey.*

*So may God use this book for HIS intended purpose and may I be obedient until the end.*

*Beth*

# Acknowledgments

I want to first and foremost thank the Lord for trusting me with this project. I have been blessed by being Your vessel to write this book. May You be glorified in this endeavor.

I would like to thank my husband, David, who treats me better than I deserve.

Thanks to my good friend Deb, who read my manuscript many times and provided valuable insight and encouragement. I could not have done this without you.

Pastor Bob, thank you for encouraging me to keep going and holding me accountable.

Thank you to Bethany, who used her God-given ability to polish this book and make it worthy of the reader's time and expense.

*Dear Friend,*

*I just heard of your recent breast cancer diagnosis and wanted to reach out to you immediately.*

*First, I want to tell you that I am so sorry that you are going through this. It could quite possibly be the hardest thing you have experienced or ever will experience. There are so many challenges you will face and so many battles to fight. At some point during this journey, you will feel all alone. You may already.*

*I am sending this letter along with my journal in the hope I can provide you some comfort. You are not alone. Let me share my experience with you—my pain, my triumphs, and my revelations—and together we will find a way through the loneliness, pain, and fear you are experiencing right now.*

*Second, I want to tell you that there is hope, and there is help. The battle is not over. If you allow me, I will show you the way. Know that no matter how hard this gets, we are fighters and we will persevere.*

*So take my hand.*

*You may feel as if you have been blindsided—that your life has been completely upended by your diagnosis. I can certainly relate. Before the cancer, I was a wife of a kind and loving man, a pastor who loved his God and his church; an active and grateful member of my church; and a blessed and busy accountant. I was an ordinary woman with an extraordinary life. And then in a moment, life changed.*

*It all started mid-April.*

# April 17

Today was Sunday.

I had just stepped out of the shower and was drying my hair when my husband came home. He had gone over to the church early to do some last-minute sermon preparations before coming home for breakfast and to see me for just a moment before heading back to start his Sunday morning routine.

As was his usual custom, he came up behind me and kissed my neck. As always, he couldn't resist cupping my breasts. I always loved that about my David, the tenderness and love he expressed in that gesture. Except this time was different.

He felt a hard knot on the left side of one of my breasts.

Fear filled me right away, because the area was very sore. I am still surprised I hadn't felt how tender the knot was before. I put my fear aside for the moment and told David we should just focus on today and not worry about the what-ifs. So we did. The morning went on, and we went to church as we would on any other Sunday. David preached a powerful sermon, and I was so proud of him.

We didn't talk about the lump on the way home. I think neither of us wanted to express our fears to the other. Instead, we stayed deep in our own thoughts. Later, David told me he was in denial. All he could think was, *Not my wife; it can't be.* But at the same time, he strongly believed God was in absolute control of our lives.

*So, my dear friend, when the lump was found, we didn't talk about it. Neither of us knew what to say, and we were trying to protect each other. I felt as though there was a great war going on between good and evil, and I honestly wasn't sure how it was going to end. So we remained silent.*

## April 18

I was troubled as I got ready for work. I kept telling myself to be patient, to wait and see what the doctor said. But I think I was already preparing for the worst.

Experience has taught me to focus on Scripture when I am afraid like this. When I stopped to calm my mind, a verse came to mind: "Surely God is my salvation, I will trust and not be afraid, The Lord, the Lord, is my strength and my song" (Isaiah 12:2). It helped a little.

The doctor's office was not open until 8:00 a.m., so at 8:01, I was on the phone. Thankfully, they had a cancellation for 1:30 the same day, so I took it. I couldn't wait another day to know what was going on.

Dr. Renata has been my family physician for the last seven years, and I love and trust her with my life. Dr. Renata did the exam and was very pleased that my breast was sore. She felt confident it was just an infected duct. She gave me antibiotics, and just to be sure, she scheduled me for a mammogram.

*I am glad my doctor took every precaution. If you're ever in a situation where you don't feel the doctors are listening or that they aren't doing everything possible, don't be afraid to speak up for yourself! You are your best, and at times possibly your only, advocate. Get a second, third, or fourth opinion.*

*Be assertive. It's your life, your body, your health, your future.*

## April 21

I was at the hospital for my mammogram today when a lady sat down beside me and offered me some kind, comforting words. I guess I must have looked scared. My mind was full with all the stories you hear from other women like how bad a mammogram hurt and how they squeezed your breast like a pancake. After childbirth and gravity had done their jobs, my breasts already looked like pancakes.

What next? Crepes, anyone?

During the mammogram, they took numerous slides of the area in question and then decided to get an ultrasound while I was there. The nurse who performed the ultrasound was very nice and, as a professional, would not tell me anything. But moments later, she stepped out and came back in with the doctor from the breast center. It is never good when the doctor comes in and looks at the ultrasound. I questioned the doctor to try to get a sense of the problem, but all the doctor would say was that it looked "worrisome."

"Worrisome." What could that mean? Worrisome takes on a whole new meaning when they are talking about your breast.

The doctor wanted to perform a biopsy right after lunch. I decided to call David and see what he thought about it. He admittedly had some misgivings. He said he had read that cutting into a cancerous mass could sometimes cause the cancer to spread to other areas. We prayed about it, and although he was still unsure, I decided to go ahead.

He said it was my decision in the end, and I needed answers. If I had a time bomb in me, I wanted to know what I was dealing with. And a biopsy seemed like the only way to get more information.

The doctor made a small incision and inserted what looked and sounded like nail clippers. She told me not to flinch when the sound went off. But that is difficult, because if someone is snipping inside your breast and you hear it, your mind expects to feel it each time. Thankfully, I didn't feel anything. Afterward, the nurse held hard pressure to my breast for a long time. It felt like I couldn't breathe. Maybe that was her pressure, or maybe it was my anxiety. They told me I would have the results tomorrow.

## April 22

When I woke up this morning, I had a voice mail. I guess I slept through the phone ringing. It was Dr. Renata, and she wanted me to come in and see her. And to bring David this time, too.

I immediately felt something was not right. It can't be good when the doctor suggests I bring my husband with me.

I wasn't sure if we had time before we left town; we were heading to a wedding in Eureka Springs, Arkansas. David said we needed to make the time, and five minutes later, we were on the road to see Dr. Renata.

Wow, I could feel the tension as we sat in the waiting room. Time ticked by so slowly, it was almost painful. Two hours passed, and we were still waiting.

I let the receptionist know we had to leave. As we were picking up our stuff, the receptionist asked us to stay a little while longer, and she would get Dr. Renata. So we stood there nervously while she went to get my doctor.

When Dr. Renata showed us to an office, I sat down, but David continued to stand. She tried to break the tension a bit and asked if he could hear from "up there." (You see, Dr. Renata is five foot one, and David is six foot seven, so there was a bit of a difference.)

Once David sat down next to me, the mood in the room got serious. Dr. Renata sat right in front of me, knee to knee, and took hold of both my hands. Somehow, I already knew what she was going to say.

And unfortunately, I was right.

"It is cancer."

So that is what "worrisome" looks like.

The C word.

She gave me a hug before David and I left. We sat in the car, just being quiet for a little bit. My mind was and still is a bit of a jumble.

Cancer.

On the way to Eureka Springs, we decided not to say anything about the cancer at the wedding and just focus on the happy event. I have to admit, though, it is ironic how we were at a wedding, watching the couple take their vows and committing to a long and wonderful future with each other. And there David and I sat, not knowing how long our future together was going to be.

One question was on repeat in me the whole time: *Is the cancer going to win?*

The wedding was beautiful. The flowers seemed more colorful and fragrant than I ever remembered. The sun shone more brightly. The hugs and smiles from family were more meaningful than ever.

But it didn't change what I had heard this morning.

My life has changed in an instant.

*In an instant, your life has changed also, but I want to say that it doesn't mean that it has to be for the worse. God is still in control, through the good and the bad. Never give up hope. Life can actually be better than it was before. That may be impossible to believe, but keep reading and keep believing. Stay strong!*

I called Mom and Dad. I tried to play it off like it was no big deal, just a minor setback, and I would keep them informed. We honestly haven't been close in so long. I felt it was the right thing to do to call them, but I really didn't want to deal with relationship issues today.

Today, the day I was diagnosed with cancer.

Next, I called Julie, my dear friend. Julie and I met in Dallas at a conference. When I think back on it now, I know it was a divine appointment. We both work in Tulsa on the same street, in the same professions; we both have daughters named Heather; we both have ex-husbands named Bob; we both struggle with our weight. Needless to say, we bonded instantly. Julie had breast cancer six years ago. So when I called her, she knew the feeling of being just diagnosed, and she just listened. She was quiet and let me talk. It was so nice! I know I rambled, but she just let me. What a gift. When I told her I had the big C, she said she saw a saying once about Christ being the Big C and cancer being a little c.

I just love Julie.

Next was Kelly. Pastor Sam and Kelly minister to a local church. David and I had met them when David was between ministries. We were close for a while, but when David accepted the preaching position at Zafra Church of Christ, we started to grow apart. She said she was sorry to hear about the cancer, I asked to be put on the prayer chain, and that was it. We hung up.

I was very disappointed with the whole conversation. Kelly is selfish; she even admits to being selfish. And the conversation was not about her, so she didn't have much interest. It made me realize how important good friends are. Especially with what I am facing now.

*My prayer is that all of your friends will stand by you. That they will be supportive and will have your back. I have read testimonials that others have had a great amount of support.*

Then I called Cindy from the office and decided to wait until Monday to tell my bosses, DJ and Butch. Cindy is wonderful. She works two days a week and is such a blessing to me. (Her husband and DJ are best friends, and her husband told DJ about the cancer before I had a chance, although I didn't know that at the time.)

## April 25

On my way to work today, I flipped on the radio, something I never do. I love my solitude, but today I couldn't stand the quiet. I turned on the local Christian radio station, and a song called "Hear My Heart" by Sherry Easter came on. I have never heard the song before. I did some looking and found that Sherry wrote it while she was going through breast cancer. God knew what I needed to hear. The words are powerful. She talks about how hard it is and how she doesn't know if she can go on. She needs God to understand how she feels. She needs God to hear her heart. She needs God to know her fears when she has no words.

This song was perfect, because it said everything I was feeling but couldn't say at the time.

It was a Monday morning, and Butch was the first to arrive. I went into his office to give him the news, but he told me he already knew and so did DJ. I was really surprised.

He told me that DJ had been freaking out all weekend trying to figure out what he was going to do. Considering I do all the accounting for the company and no one else knows the software, DJ was pretty worried. When he showed up at the office later, he was already talking about bringing someone in to learn my job. That freaked me out. Once DJ and I had a chance to talk, we both calmed down. I really wish I had been the one to tell him.

I work with some really great men. They are very respectful of me, and they watch their language. I appreciate all of them so much.

I e-mailed my friend Deb. She is hard of hearing, so our conversations are best by e-mail. I really appreciate Deb. I can write two brief sentences, and she totally gets how I am feeling. And then she takes the time to write me a book back. Today was no exception. So grateful for her!

I had an appointment this afternoon to see a surgeon, Dr. Taylor. David went with me.

On the way, we talked a little bit about it all. David told the guys at his work that I have cancer, and one guy told my husband that it was his fault, that I fall under his umbrella of protection, and since I have cancer, that means he has sin in his life that needs dealt with. First of all, I can't believe anyone would believe that or tell someone else that. *That it is my husband's fault.* What bologna.

*"His disciples asked him, 'Rabbi, who sinned, this man or his parents, that he was born blind?' 'Neither this man nor his parents sinned,' said Jesus, 'but this happened so that the works of God might be displayed in his life'" (John 9:2-3).*

*Okay, here is where I want to tell you, you will need a thick skin to walk through this. People are going to be insensitive and downright thoughtless. There will be outrageous, disgusting comments made to you and about you. It's wrong, yes. But it's going to happen. You can waste your energy being upset when it does, or you can prepare yourself to let the comments and cruelty slide off your back and not bring you down.*

*Father in heaven, I pray that You will protect my friend's heart and shut the mouths of mean people. And, Father, I pray that she will not have to go through the same cruelty that I had to experience. Please help her focus on Your goodness and Your healing. Amen.*

David and I held hands while we waited in Dr. Taylor's office. I felt like I was holding on for dear life. We didn't have to wait long to be seen, which I was grateful for, and when Dr. Taylor entered, he had already looked at the films and biopsy. He felt like we had caught the cancer early.

The technical term for my cancer is DCIS, which stands for ductal carcinoma in situ. *Ductal* means it is in the milk ducts, *carcinoma* simply means cancer, and *in situ* means it hasn't spread to any other areas yet.

Dr. Taylor said it was the best kind of breast cancer to have, if someone was going to have cancer. For some odd reason, that thought is very comforting to me, even now. He recommended a lumpectomy, which is a surgical procedure that removes only the affected area and a margin around it, to make sure I'm free of any bad tissue. The surgery is outpatient. The specimen will then be sent to the lab to be tested. We need a clear margin of unaffected tissue all the way around the lump, which is called "clean margins."

He did say I would need radiation after the surgery. But then I would be cancer-free, so no big deal, right?

But it did seem like a big deal. He was going to remove part of my breast. But I was very thankful they would not have to remove my entire breast. I have felt ever since I was young, that I would never have any body part removed. I am not sure where that came from, but it is a strong conviction.

I called Mom and Dad, and they agreed to put me on the prayer list at church. I called my friend Julie, and I called Kelly. Once again, Julie was supportive and Kelly was not.

I was reminded of a sermon I heard years ago that really left an impression on me. So I called Pastor Sam, who had given the message, and asked if he would send me his notes again. I read them many times already. I pray I can use this lesson from God and this lesson from cancer to change my life.

## "Writing Your life Story"

Decisions you make will have a huge impact on your story . . . and you. Right now, you get to choose what story you tell. Everything you're doing right now, every decision you make, will eventually be a part of your story, and you've got to decide what story you want to tell . . . I know you want to be able to tell your whole story . . . You want that story to be consistent and true to what you believe and understand . . . You don't want to have to hide anything or try to forget it.

You've always got to remember, with each choice, with each decision you are faced with, there are consequences, both good and bad, awaiting your choice.

*I don't think I will ever forget that sermon; I want my story to make a difference. I don't want to die and it not matter that I ever lived. I think about dying sometimes. It is not fear of where I am going but the painful process of getting there that I worry about. There is nothing like a life-threatening illness to cause some self-reflection.*

## April 26

Dealing with insurance now. My policy includes a onetime payout upon first diagnosis of cancer. I called Dr. Renata's office to fax over a copy of my lab work so I could get the process going.

It came later that day. Down in the bottom left of the report, it clearly stated that I had had cancer in my right breast in the past. That was absolutely not true, and the statement would cost me $20,000 if it were. So I called the lab, and they said there wasn't anything they could do about it because that was the information they had received from Dr. Renata's office.

Somewhat frustrated, I called Dr. Renata's office, and they said they would look into it. That wasn't very promising. So I called the lab back. Apparently, the process was somewhat complicated. They said Dr. Renata would need to fill out a form, and then I would have to go to a board for review to contest the charge. If the board approved, then the item would be removed from my pathology report.

The nurse's name that I spoke to was Kathy. It turns out she is a breast cancer survivor, and she said she would do everything she could to help me. I could see the finger of God in getting her on the phone this time.

So Kathy sent the form over to Dr. Renata's office, and Dr. Renata's office confirmed that they had gotten it. So now I just had to wait.

*My friend, no matter how big or how many obstacles are put in your path, FIGHT! Do not let the problems stop you. Keep moving. Keep fighting.*

## April 27

Sylvia stopped by the office to talk to me. She works just down the road from me, and I know her from church. She was greatly troubled. She said she had heard about my cancer but that the church had not put me on the prayer chain. When she mentioned my name for prayer, Pastor Sam said that wasn't to be made public, that I am a very private person. Which I didn't understand, because I had called Kelly and asked to be put on the prayer chain. So that evening, I asked David to give Pastor Sam a call, which he did. I figured it was just a miscommunication.

## April 28

I followed up with Dr. Renata's office. Two days had passed, but no progress had been made on the form.

I was pretty frustrated with the whole thing, so I got online to distract myself. There is a woman that does an alternative to yoga. She always asks for prayer requests, so today I decided to respond. I told her what was going on.

She replied almost immediately and sent me some Scriptures to look up, and she asked if she could call me. I said, "Of course," and she called a couple of hours later. First, we discussed the Scriptures she had sent. Then she said, "If you want to be healed, all you need to do is believe that you are healed." And she asked me, "Do you believe?" I told her I would have to think about it, and we hung up.

*Here's the thing. I don't believe someone can heal himself or herself by simply believing. I believe God will heal me if He chooses to and will not heal me if He chooses not to. My life is in God's hands, not mine. God uses many different methods to heal someone. And I take comfort in knowing that the God of the universe, the Creator of heaven and earth, has my life in His hands. Not only my life but the cancer policy also.*

## April 29

Called Dr. Renata's office—the form had not been completed. I made an appointment for the afternoon, hoping to make something happen. When I saw Dr. Renata, she didn't know anything about me waiting for a form. And no one even knew where the form was. I wanted to scream. I was putting my life in their hands, and they couldn't even take care of a piece of paper.

I called Kathy, and she faxed it over right away. Dr. Renata filled it out while I waited and personally called the lab to ensure that everything would be taken care of and that the form would be sufficient. So I left feeling a bit better, having completed part of the process. Now I just needed a revised pathology report. Kathy said to give her until Monday.

*I believe God sent the lady in the waiting room and Kathy in pathology into my life to help me. God knew what help I would need before I even needed it. Thank You, Lord.*

## May 2

I called Kathy, and she said the pathologist that signed my original form was gone for two weeks and the pathologist on duty didn't want to change another doctor's report, so I would have to wait. Waiting is so hard. Every minute seems like an hour, and every day seems like a week, and every week feels like a year.

Sylvia stopped by the office again and said that Pastor Sam still refused to put me on the prayer list. She was visibly upset about it. I tried to encourage her, but it was kind of difficult since I didn't understand what was going on myself. I think one of the hardest things about cancer is how my "friends" have acted.

Instead of dwelling on something I had no control over, I decided to look up Christian comedians on YouTube. I laughed my head off for quite a while.

*Proverbs 17:22 says, "A joyful heart is good medicine, but a crushed spirit dries up the bones."*

*I believe laughter and attitude have a lot to do with our ability to fight this cancer. Try to find things to laugh at. Look up online Christian comedians, tell jokes, laugh out loud, and try to get others to join in. Think back to an easier time when you laughed often.*

*What was it that tickled you? Find that thing and do it again. Go to a park and watch people. People are funny. Go to a funny movie. Spend time with upbeat people.*

*Q: What kind of bees produces milk?*
*A: Boobies!*
*Ha-ha.*

*I read nine benefits of laughter therapy on the Cancer Treatment Centers of America's website that I would like to share with you.*

1. *Boosts the immune system and circulatory system*
2. *Enhances oxygen intake*
3. *Stimulates the heart and lungs*
4. *Relaxes the muscles throughout the body*
5. *Triggers the release of endorphins*
6. *Eases digestion/soothes stomach aches*
7. *Relieves pain*
8. *Balances blood pressure*
9. *Improves mental functions (alertness, memory, creativity)*

*See? You need to laugh!*

*I read in one of my many cancer books a little story called "Attitude."*

*There was once a woman who woke up one morning, looked in the mirror, and noticed she had only three hairs on her head.*

*"Well," she said, "I think I will braid my hair today."*

*So she did, and she had a wonderful day. The next day she woke up, looked in the mirror, and saw that she had only two hairs on her head.*

*"Hmm," she said. "I think I'll part my hair down the middle today. So she did, and she had a grand day.*

*The next day she woke up, looked in the mirror, and noticed that she had only one hair on her head.*

*"Well," she said, "today I'm going to wear my hair in a ponytail." So she did, and she had her best day, so far!*

*The next day she woke up, looked in the mirror, and noticed there wasn't a single hair on her head.*

*"Yahoo!" she exclaimed. "I don't have to fix my hair today!"*

*Bottom line: attitude is everything.*

*As the saying goes, "The kind of life you will have isn't determined by what happens to you. It's determined by your reaction to what happens to you."*

*Author unknown*

*How is your attitude? Are you doing okay?*

## May 3-5

David was out of town at the Kiamichi Men's Clinic that is held every year at Christ 40 Acres (a camp close to Zafra in the Kiamichi Mountains). He was responsible for the preacher boy contest. There were seven boys prepared to preach that week, and David had gotten many Bible colleges to donate tuition for the top three winners. I believe David was torn about going, but I insisted since there was nothing he could do here. And the clinic was important to him. While down there, he had some close friends pray for me. One pastor that he talked to recommended a naturopathic doctor that he liked in Fort Smith. Although having a doctor in Fort Smith is not practical because of the distance, the recommendation did get David thinking about finding a naturopath here in Tulsa.

I got a call from Dr. Taylor. He said he saw a spot on some of my recent films that he wanted to look at and asked me to come into his office.

I always talk to David in the morning and at night when he is out of town to touch base with him and to feel close to him. I took the opportunity to bring up Dr. Taylor's call. I had scheduled my appointment for the next day. David felt bad for not being there with me, but it was okay; I understood.

But when I arrived at the office for the appointment the next day, David was there waiting, and he had flowers. I was so thrilled! I still can't believe he drove all the way home just for the appointment. And afterward, he had another four hours to get back in time for the evening session. He loves me so very much. I am very blessed.

The appointment was brief. Dr. Taylor mentioned that there was an area of concern that he wanted to check on.

Thankfully, it was not a mass! It was fluid, which he removed. He seemed very encouraged by that fact. I was encouraged as well, and even more so that David was there with me.

*Friend, there were many times during my cancer journey that my husband could not relate to me or understand, but this time he did the absolutely perfect thing. I am so blessed to have this moment to hold onto. Just being there showed he cared.*

## May 6

I got the pathology report. It was correct this time. Yeah! I immediately sent it off to the insurance company. It feels so good to have that finally resolved.

## May 11

I found a naturopathic doctor in Tulsa, and he works days at the cancer treatment center. I feel really fortunate to have found him. Another divine appointment. Thank You, Jesus.

# May 17

First appointment with Dr. Kendall, the naturopath. He told me about a couple of items I could get at the cancer center pharmacy to help with healing after my surgery. One item was for sugar control, which apparently helps the healing process; the other was called Arnica. The container has a twist bottom so you can turn it until three tiny little pellets drop down, and then you remove the cap and pour them into your mouth. They are to be kept under your tongue until they dissolve. It is important to not touch them. Arnica is used to prevent excess fluid buildup, stimulate respiration, ease pain, and reduce swelling. I'm looking forward to seeing how it works.

Dr. Kendall was so helpful. He spent the entire evening with David and me, listening and providing support. This was a very timely appointment since my lumpectomy is in two days.

I haven't given much thought to the upcoming surgery. I think I am in denial.

I do think I will go home and take some pictures of my breast. A before and after picture. I've heard some woman get a plaster replica made before surgery. Interesting, but no.

*I think it is important to pursue all areas when it comes to your healing. Consider alternative medicine to supplement the traditional medicine. Search out ways to help you heal emotionally and spiritually. Consider acupuncture for relaxation. Search the web for information.*

*I have two three-inch notebooks filled with information I collected. Again, you are your own best advocate. Research, research, research!*

## May 18

A check from the cancer policy—$20,000—arrived today. I want to be very careful how it is spent.

*My friend, I have been very blessed with great health insurance. My employer also picks up the deductible. I don't know your financial situation, but the bills adding up can add a lot pressure. Pressure that you don't need. In many states, there are a great number of resources available for assistance. This would be a good job for your caregiver to research and fill out applications for you. There are cleaning agencies who will clean your house while you are taking chemo. There is transportation and prescription assistance also, and much more.*

## May 19

Lumpectomy is scheduled for today. I need to be at the hospital at 6:30 a.m. Heather and Leaha, my daughters, have taken off from work to be there at the hospital and to wait with David. Will write more after it is all over.

Well, it's over with now.

The mood was festive with my daughters there, and it really felt like this was going to be easy.

I was supposed to take everything off and put on a gown. There was no way I was going to take my panties off though. I can be pretty modest at times. And since they were not operating down there, I didn't see any reason.

Later I found out it is because sometimes, under anesthesia, a person will leak a little. I didn't care. If someone was going to cut a piece of my breast off, I wanted to be as comfortable as possible. Silly, I know.

The operation went well. Dr. Taylor talked to David while I was in recovery and said that he thought he got it all, that he was positive overall. Anesthesia made me nauseous, so they kept me a little longer, and I don't remember anything until I woke up back in the room and they were giving me some ginger ale to drink. When David told me what Dr. Taylor said, I was ecstatic and thankful that it was over.

My surgery was on a Thursday and David had to leave Friday, so he called his cousin to come over and stay with me. She never showed up, but I was fine. I just rested and stayed home.

## May 21

Our thirteenth wedding anniversary. David had a wedding to perform, and I was home recuperating. Not the best way to celebrate. But thank God the cancer is gone.

*How do I say this? I should have fought for the sanctity of our marriage, even while I was fighting for my life. I didn't, and I regret that. I encourage you to learn from my mistake and stand by your convictions. Fight for what is right. My husband should have been home for our anniversary, and he should have been home when I was recuperating. It is not David's fault. I am absolutely sure I told him it was okay instead of saying no.*

## May 23

Monday morning and I am back at work. It is truly amazing what doctors can do with God's help.

## May 25

I turned forty-seven, and my left breast is smaller than my right, but the minor setback in my life is over.

*Let me explain what a minor setback meant to me. I work at my job, I work for fun, I work at helping others, I enjoy work. This was a minor setback because the surgery was on Thursday and I was back to work on Monday.*

*As far as life, this was huge. This was no minor setback. A part of my breast was missing, and cancer had taken it.*

I found an illustration online that I really liked and I ran right out to the store and bought two jars and some beads.

The first jar is filled with beads that represent a day of your life. So each day you take one out and put it in your pocket or on your desk as a reminder that when this day is gone, it cannot be redeemed. So what am I going to do with it? Don't waste it. It is precious and don't let one day become two and seven and thirty and 365 without making a difference. At the end of the day, it goes into the other jar. It is gone.

It is a great illustration for me since I am so visual, and it helps me stay focused and not lose track of time.

*I am writing my life story. Do you remember what Pastor Sam talked about? That every day, we are writing our life story, and if I am not careful, it becomes a day of work, anger, and time lost without ever reaching out to anyone.*

*What will your life story be? What has it been so far? Are you proud or ashamed of it? It is not too late to start another chapter and change whatever path you have been on. Some people don't get an opportunity to stop and consider life. You have been given a blessing in disguise. I know it is hard to think about it like that right now, but when you are ready, give it some thought.*

## May 26

Tammy called me from Dr. Taylor's office and wanted me to come in to see Dr. Taylor this afternoon. I wasn't worried and didn't even call David to tell him. David had taken off enough work already. They got me right into the exam room when I arrived. Dr. Taylor looked concerned. When I saw his face, I wished I had called David. My heart sunk. I knew this was not good.

The pathology report came back. No clear margins. When the surgeon removes the cancer, he also removes an extra area around the lump. That way he knows that they got it all. In this case, he got no clear margins. Nowhere around the lump was cancer-free. Nowhere!

He needed to perform another lumpectomy.

This time he would make sure he took enough area so that he got it all. He was actually surprised that *no* area was clear.

I was so shocked and confused. I remember him saying he felt good about the surgery, and I never, for one minute, thought I still had cancer.

Why hadn't I called David? Why hadn't any alarms gone off in my head when the nurse called? I know why. Because I never for one minute thought I still had cancer.

I went straight home and told David everything that had happened, saying that I would need another surgery.

He had a lot of questions I couldn't answer. I felt attacked and lonely. He was clearly upset, and so was I. I wanted comfort, and he wanted answers. It was awful.

*The men in our life really just want to fix things. When they can't, they often lash out. David was not mad at me. He was just frustrated. But it still caused a wedge between us. What I really needed was for him to hold me. Try to understand that even when you are disappointed, confused, and hurt that our caregivers are struggling too. It is harder to watch a loved one be in pain and suffer than it is being the one who suffers.*

*This area of contention between us didn't have to happen. All I had to do was call him when Dr. Taylor requested I come in, and he would have been there. My friend, it is important for your caregiver to be with you at every appointment. You never know what the doctor will say, how you will feel, or if you will remember what is said. Lean on that support. You need it, and they need you too.*

## May 27

The Friday before Memorial Day weekend, I had to tell my bosses that I still had cancer and that I needed another surgery. It was not fun. I had reassured DJ that this was no big deal, and honestly, now I wasn't so sure.

My next surgery is scheduled for next Thursday. David was in Zafra, and I didn't feel like I had the energy to drive the four hours to go down there. So I spent the weekend alone, scared, and confused.

I realize it wasn't the best thing to do, but I used the time to create my bucket list.

**Bucket List**

1. Solve world hunger.
2. Go on an Alaskan cruise. (David said if I was a five-year survivor or only had six months to live, we could go—not the most sensitive comment.)
3. Focus on relationships.
4. Get my affairs in order.

5. Try sushi. (Odd, I know, but the guys have sushi Friday all the time. Any day of the week can be sushi Friday, and I have always wanted to go.)
6. Write letters to my girls, all nine of them: Heather, Leaha, Judith, Deborah, Terra, Alex, Haley, Tori, and Nicole. (Heather and Leaha are my biological children, Judith and Deborah are my children by marriage, and Terra, Alex, Haley, Tori, and Nicole are my children through church relationships.)
7. Ride a Harley.

*My friend, may I remind us what Philippians 4:7-8 says:*

*And the peace of God, which transcends all understanding, will guard your hearts and your minds in Christ Jesus. Finally, whatever is true, whatever is noble, whatever is right, whatever is pure, whatever is lovely, whatever is admirable—if anything is excellent or praiseworthy—think about such things.*

*It is not what I did, but it is good advice.*

## May 29

I decided to attend Collinsville Christian Church this Sunday. I have been there before, and I felt like I really needed to be there today. The sermon was exceptional, and I went forward after the sermon to ask for prayer. Pastor Bob had everyone come forward and lay hands on me while he prayed.

It was just what I needed.

# June 2

This feels like déjà vu. We arrived at the hospital at 6:00 a.m. and have been waiting for Dr. Taylor to remove more of my breast. Even though this is the same hospital, David and I can't believe the difference. I was put into a room at the end of the hall, and hours later, we are still waiting.

David actually went to find someone because we thought they had forgotten us. Finally, they came in, started an IV, and gave me a gown to put on. Heather came to sit with David, but Leaha couldn't get off work this time.

Dr. Taylor came in and we prayed together. He patted my shoulder and tried to reassure me. His plan is to take a generous sample of tissue so he could get clear margins this time. At this point, I thought I would just wait and see. Here we go again.

Surgery went well. The nausea was worse this time, but I made it through. Now we wait, *again*, for the pathology report.

*I pray you are more patient than I am. Isaiah 40:31 says,*

*But those who hope on the Lord will renew their strength; they will soar on wings like eagles, they will run and not grow weary, they will walk and not faint.*

# June 6

After work, I went to a breast cancer support group. No one besides the leader was there. The instructor gave me a good opportunity to ask questions, but I was looking for connection and fellowship. I wanted to hug someone who had been through the storm and had survived. I wanted to draw strength from her.

*My friend, I wish I could tell you that I turned to God. I didn't. Not on this day. Instead, I wallowed in self-pity.*

*I cannot express the loneliness I felt when I reached out for comfort and couldn't find it. I don't understand why this was my journey, except that my abandonment helped me to eventually draw closer to God. God has promised to never leave us or forsake us. That is a promise. He never said that people wouldn't.*

*Dear God,*

*I want to pray for my friend because she may experience this awful aloneness and abandonment. Please bring Your comfort and presence to my friend right now as she reads this and every time she needs it. Hug her and stay with her. Give her a peace that passes all understanding. With You by her side, she will never be alone. Thank You for that. And thank you for staying with me, even when I couldn't feel You there. Father, please send her friends who will walk this path with her. In Jesus Name. Amen.*

# June 8

Tammy called and wants me to come in and see Dr. Taylor. I said, "No, you just put him on the phone and tell me right now. I am *not* coming in." I couldn't deal with the whole process again. I just needed to know.

A little while later, Dr. Taylor came on the phone, and he said the pathology report had come back with *no* clear margins. He didn't understand why, because he had taken a generous portion of tissue.

So I took a deep breath and asked, "What now?"

He said I would need a mastectomy. He wanted me to see an oncologist first, and then we would schedule it.

Talk about overload. I didn't understand, and I was so frustrated and upset by the news. I needed to talk to David, who I knew would have even more questions than I did, so I suggested Dr. Taylor call that evening so we could all talk about this together. He agreed.

Dr. Taylor called about eight in the evening, and we talked for an hour and a half. David got all his questions answered. Truthfully, I couldn't really absorb any of it.

What happened to "no big deal" and "the best cancer to have"?

What a joke.

My breast was going to be completely removed, or so they were saying. I never wanted any body part removed. I feel like I would die first before I let that happen.

David didn't like the way I was talking; he was really struggling hearing me talk that way. I couldn't help it. It is how I feel.

He said he is too close to the situation to be objective. David's way of coping is by giving me Scriptures whenever I say anything. He always wants me to be positive and upbeat. I feel like he just doesn't let me feel what I am going through.

I wish I could just grieve and go through it. I wish I had someone who would just listen instead of telling me how to feel or how not to feel.

So here goes . . . The doctor wants to remove my breast in order to save my life, and I would rather die than have my breast removed.

*My Friend, sometimes my journal focused on the negative. There was good also.*

*God brought Sheila into my life through her brother Mike, who I work with. Sheila started e-mailing me with wonderful words of encouragement, and she brought a gift by the office. Next, she told her mom about me, and a little while later, she too was sending cards. What a blessing from people I didn't even know!*

*I received many flowers and cards from the ladies at Zafra Church of Christ, from all three of my bosses, and from my friend Jerri Ann. So, my friend, I want to encourage you to look for these shining stars in the darkness. These were my angels that God sent with flesh on. He will send you some too.*

## June 14

David called the mental health center associated with a hospital here in Tulsa and made me an appointment. I really wasn't too keen on going, but I respect my husband and trust he is doing what he can to help me. My appointment is with Dr. Baxter, a nun at the clinic.

I got there, and honestly, I was a little intimidated by the habit on her head and her dress. I am not sure why. I guess because I really wasn't sure about being there in the first place.

She took me back to her office, and after we sat down, the first thing she said was, "I will not see you." I was confused because if she wouldn't see me, why had I taken off work and why was I sitting in her office. And she kept repeating it: "I will not see you. I will not see you."

So finally, I got up my nerve, said, "Okay," and got up to leave.

She stopped me, saying it all hit too close to home for her and that she couldn't be objective about her counseling. She mentioned another counselor, Diane, who could counsel me but was not available today. She said that Diane would call me.

I left rejected, confused, and mad.

I never heard from Diane, and it doesn't matter. I was *never* going back to that place.

David was angry when I told him about it. He doesn't get angry often, but he was that time. I didn't know it at the time, but he called his brother Joe to talk to him about it. Let me just say that if David calls on brother power, he is upset.

*How well you do in this crisis will be directly related to the amount of social support you receive. What are you doing when a door closes?*

*Let me say it again. How well you do in this crisis will be directly related to the amount of social support you receive. Receive, not give but receive. When your husband doesn't understand, find someone else to talk to; when a church shuts the door, find another church; when a counselor refuses to see you, find another counselor. It is draining to keep trying, but it is valuable to your health.*

## June 22

I have my appointment with Dr. Andrews, the oncologist, today. If you ever want to see death, go to an oncologist's office. It is much worse than a funeral home. Sit in the waiting room with all the people that have no hair, no energy, and no strength. It is not fun. Not fun at all.

I liked Dr. Andrews. He offered me hope. I can't explain it, but there is something empowering about having someone listen and take time to really be there in the moment, understanding what you're going through. I felt like I had someone on my team who really cared about me, and that felt good.

## June 23

I called Tammy and scheduled the mastectomy for June 30. Dr. Taylor told me to see the oncologist and then have the surgery, so that is what I am doing. I called Mom and Dad, and they said they were coming down.

I didn't argue. I am glad they are coming.

I don't think I ever consciously made the decision to go forward with the surgery. I just acted, or maybe *reacted*. Julie said my thinking about not having the mastectomy was a lack of faith. She said it actually made her mad when I talked like that. Whatever happened to just listening and letting me vent? Those days were gone apparently.

Why does everyone think they know what is best for me? I am the only one who is going to suffer the consequences of my decision. Shouldn't I be the one to choose without judgment?

## June 27

Mom and Dad left Ohio for the trip to Oklahoma. It is a two-day trip by car, but Dad has had heart problems in the past and they just wanted to take it easy on the way down. They might stop and rest.

## June 28

Dr. Taylor called. He was surprised to see me on the surgery schedule. He said he wasn't ready.

I don't understand! He said, "See the oncologist, and then have surgery."

He said he wants to schedule an MRI to see what is going on before he does surgery. The only problem with scheduling an MRI is that it needs to be between day eight and ten of my cycle. So I have to wait to start my period before the MRI can be scheduled.

Well, there goes the plan. I immediately called Mom and Dad. They were two hours out.

Mom and Dad were at the house by the time I got home from work. They decided to stay the weekend and then went back to Ohio. Who knows when the surgery will be scheduled now?

# July 13

My mom's birthday and the day of my MRI. They are scanning both breasts because Dr. Taylor wanted to get more data. He really felt confident that he could get all the cancer with the first surgery, and then was totally confident he could get it all with the second surgery. So now that neither happened the way he planned, he is second-guessing himself and the information that he had. Why, oh Lord? How did I get here, and why am I here? I am so confused.

He said he would call me the same day with the results.

Since I was at work, I asked Butch, my boss, if he would listen in when Dr. Taylor called. Sometimes, emotions take over and it is hard to remember. He said he would, which I was thankful for.

Dr. Taylor called. Butch was listening for the phone call, so he came into my office and shut the door. The results were inconclusive. He wants to perform the mastectomy on the left breast, then wait three months, do another scan on the right breast, then do a second mastectomy if necessary.

I can't believe it. I'm in total shock.

I asked Dr. Taylor about not having the mastectomy at all, and Butch, sitting there with his head down, moaned. It was a sound both of fear and compassion. But he didn't say anything. I really appreciated Butch's support. Not many bosses would have done that. I work with some incredible guys.

*You have searched me, Lord, and you know me.*

*You know when I sit and when I rise; you perceive my thoughts from afar. You discern my going out and my lying down; you are familiar with all my ways. Before a word is on my tongue, you, Lord, know it completely. You hem me in behind and before, and you lay your hand upon me . . . . Your eyes saw my unformed body; all the days ordained for me were written in your book before one of them came to be. Psalm 139:1-5, 16*

## July 19

Everyone keeps telling me, "Get a second opinion. Get a second opinion." So I called Dr. Smith. She is a breast specialist in my area, but she works out of another network. My insurance won't cover it, but I decided to go out of network for a second opinion. I might as well at this point.

## July 20

Dr. Smith did a full exam, looked at all the data, and confirmed that a mastectomy was necessary. I wanted to know what she thought about having a double mastectomy if I had one at all, just to be done with it. She talked a lot about the value of being balanced, that it would not be a bad decision if I went that way. It felt good to have her validate Dr. Taylor. I was honestly beginning to question his ability.

I told Cindy that I was thinking about not having the mastectomy at all, and she said, "You can't make me love you then die." Cindy sometimes waivers in her faith, and I couldn't show her a lack of faith.

I called Tammy and scheduled the double mastectomy for August 3. My husband was admittedly reluctant to have the second breast removed. But he deferred to my decision. He didn't buy into the idea of "value in being balanced," but he understood that I was tired and didn't want to do this again in three months.

That same day, I hired Vicky to come into the office and work with me and learn my job. I was going to be out for a full two weeks.

*Friend, I knew, as if God had spoken directly to me, that I cared more about Cindy and her salvation than my own breast. May I encourage you to find a quiet place and pray until you feel a peace about your decision. You and you alone will be faced with the consequences every day. This is your life and your health and your body, and this is your decision.*

*I don't intend to leave out my husband, because he too suffers the consequences of this decision. But David doesn't look in the mirror and see this every day. He doesn't have to worry every time he bends over that someone will see the scars, or deal with the heat from the prosthesis, or have this sickening ache when buying clothes, or feel the discomfort from the seat belt rubbing the incision. David has days where he doesn't even think about this anymore. I never have those days.*

## July 22

Cindy and I had sushi for lunch. Bucket list #5 accomplished!

I found a leather vest that had a cross, the fish symbol, and praises to God on it. It was perfect. Butch brought his Harley into the office so Cindy took pictures of me on it. I even took my top off and took a picture with the vest and my black lace bra on the bike. Bucket list #7 accomplished!

Well, at least as close to it as I will ever get.

## August 1

Mom and Dad arrive. I am so glad they came back. I'm so thankful that I didn't have to ask.

## August 2

Day before the big day, I received an e-mail that meant the entire world to me.

Beth to Deb:

Can I ask for prayer today? My attitude stinks, and my husband is suffering the wrath of Beth. Also feeling forsaken and angry at God. (Just an emotion. I know logically that it is not true, but an emotion nonetheless.) Thanks for letting me be honest.

Deb to Beth:

Dear God,

We really don't know how Adam felt when he woke up mutated without a rib, but we know that he got a wife out of it. You did not make us to be cut up and to lose our parts, and it is infuriating and frustrating when a doctor says it is our only chance for life. *So what is the deal?* You are God! Why couldn't you just take this cancer *out* without surgery and without all this pain!

Father, we are women. Breasts are important to us! And this loss is a very personal hard loss. We want to rant and rave; we want to shout and beg for a recount!

And through it all, we know that you are God. And you make decisions and choices, and because we are human, we have to live by them. So today, God, we acknowledge that you have made this choice, fully knowing how we feel and what it means to us. So, God, we lay our whole bodies at your feet. We ask you to take control of all things, so Beth will live on earth more than a short time.

Even the sacrifice of body parts is less to us than the loss of her sweet spirit.

As we lay before you, we ask for mercy and healing.

Please make her doctor rested and highly skilled. Make her nurses caring and tender. And when this healing is done, we ask that you use this experience to bring other women with cancer to you through the heart and spirit of my beloved Beth. Please turn something so crummy into something beautiful.

So today, I ask for peace and joy—a miracle only you can provide. We love you, God. Stay very, very, very close to my friend. You know how much I need her. Hold her in your loving arms and bring her comfort.

In Jesus Name, Amen.

## August 3

The morning of my double mastectomy. Wow, the room was full. Sherry and Rosie came all the way from Zafra, and Pastor Bob, Heather, Leaha, Mom, Dad, Julie, and David. It was just what I needed. Sherry is the funniest lady I know. She had all of us in stitches, and the time went fast. She kept my mind off the inevitable.

A nurse came from the nuclear medicine department to inject radioactive dye into my lymph nodes so that they glowed during surgery.

Everyone had to leave the room briefly. Dr. Taylor was going to take a few lymph nodes and test them for cancer to see if the cancer had spread. If it had, we would have to consider chemotherapy.

David was allowed back in after that was over. He kissed me. I quickly grabbed his hand and put it on my breast for one more feel before they were gone. That memory will have to last forever.

Everyone else came back in, and we laughed some more. Finally, it was time, and they wheeled me out.

I was in the hallway outside of the operating room and asked the nurse what they do with the breast tissue after pathology was done. She said she guessed they incinerated it.

I never wanted a piece of my body cut off. I would rather die.

*2 Corinthians 4:16-18 says,*

*Therefore we do not lose heart. Though outwardly we are wasting away, yet inwardly we are being renewed day by day. For our light and momentary troubles are achieving for us an eternal glory that far outweighs them all. So we fix our eyes not on what is seen, but on what is unseen. For what is seen is temporary, but what is unseen is eternal.*

Dr. Taylor said they tested the lymph nodes while I was in surgery, and they came back clear of cancer. That was great news.

I don't remember recovery. I thought I woke up in bed in my room, but Mom says I woke up on the gurney and refused to let the orderly move me, insisting on getting in the bed myself. That sounds like me; even only partly conscious, I can be strong willed and assertive.

It had been a long day for everyone, and once I made it out of recovery, everyone but Julie and David headed home.

I don't remember where David went, but at one point, Julie and I were in the room alone. I looked down my shirt, at my chest. I had done a lot of research, so I knew what to expect.

This was not it. This was gross.

I told Julie how gross it was, and she didn't understand. She just thought I meant because my breasts were gone. Actually, the doctor had left a lot of skin and fat hanging in various spots, and it looked like a lot of hills and valleys across my chest all taped up with clear plastic so I could see everything. I had four tubes coming out of my body with bulbs at the end to collect fluid.

I looked like a freak. I felt like a freak. I *was* a freak.

I slept quite a bit that day, but at one point, my precious Cindy came and visited. DJ and Butch had sent her shopping, and she brought me a Kindle, along with magazines, snacks for David, and pedicure stuff. It was the best gift basket ever. She didn't stay long, but that was okay. I was tired.

Dr. Taylor came in to see me. He sat down on the edge of the bed next to me. I asked him why it looked so gross. He said to show him, so I pulled my shirt out at the collar and he looked down my top. I think I blushed. It felt odd to have a man who was not my husband look down my top. I realize there was no breast, but that area has always been private and it seemed inappropriate. Anyway, he explained that he didn't want to cut too much skin and then not be able to pull it together to sew up. If he had, I would need skin grafts and that would be bad. Since I still had anesthesia in my system, it sounded reasonable to me.

*David and I still wonder if this was Dr. Taylor's first mastectomy. We don't know for sure, but we suspect it was. Please do your research on your doctor. I saw whatever surgeon my family doctor referred me to. I didn't ask questions. I may have suffered more than needed to as a result.*

*Dear Lord,*

*Please give my friend wisdom. Please guide her. Please be in front preparing the way for her. Lay the right questions on her heart to ask. Surround her with knowledgeable doctors. Help her to find a way to research her doctor's competence and experience. Make her path clear. Remove all obstacles.*

*Lord, she needs You now.*

## August 4

I slept well for being in a hospital bed, having nurses check on me every four hours, and noises that were unfamiliar. There was a bed in the room that David could stay in, and his presence that close gave me a lot of security.

Dr. Taylor checked in on me around eight, and I was sitting up talking. He asked how I felt, and I said I was fine and ready to go home. He said there wasn't anything more the hospital could do for me, so he was okay with me going home and would sign my discharge papers. The nurse came in and showed David and me how to take care of the drain tubes, and I headed home about ten that morning.

## August 5

Mom was helping me with my drain tubes when David came into the bathroom. He wanted to be the one to help me. He said something about not being needed and left. A little bit later, he came in to talk to me and asked if I minded if he went ahead and went to Zafra (where David ministers on the weekend). I think he felt displaced, but I also think he needed time to deal with his own loss. So I agreed and he took off.

## August 6-15

Mom and Dad took really good care of me. We had a lot of good talks, and I feel this time together was healing for our relationship. At one point, I was telling Dad about my leather vest and my picture on the Harley. I showed Dad the vest, and he said that he was jealous.

*Let me encourage you, my friend, to accept help. It is a hard thing to do, but necessary. It is a win-win situation. You get to experience humility; therefore, you develop character and your helper gets to be a blessing.*

## August 16

It was time for my follow up visit with Dr. Taylor, and I was really hopeful that he would remove my drain tubes. I was healing nicely, so he decided that yes, he would remove them. Mom got a chance to ask him about all the skin that he had not removed. I think he was a little frustrated because I had already asked him previously. He just explained that it was necessary in order to make sure he had enough skin in order to close up the incision. Since I was doing so well, he released me to go back to work and to resume driving.

Since the cancer was gone, I did not need chemotherapy or radiation. What a blessing. Dad explained that he had been praying for complete healing and God did answer his prayers, just not the way he meant it. I was saved from the agony of chemo, radiation, and was not feeling any pain from the surgery. Praise God.

Mom and Dad headed back to Ohio. I slipped the leather vest into the suitcase and asked Mom not to tell Dad.

## August 17

I went back to work. Vicky was doing some of my work for me while I was gone. She did a good job, but she also did it her way and not mine. Since I am so structured, that was really hard for me. Vicky finished the rest of the week.

This is my first day back at work, and when I get home, there is a card on my front porch. It was from Pastor Sam, apologizing for his behavior. It really made me angry. It just stirred up all the feelings of abandonment that I felt.

## August 22

Everything went back to normal for everyone except me. I really hate this skin. I had done a lot of research on what a mastectomy looked like. I had prepared myself, but not for this. This is deformed. There is a photographer from New York that published a book of many different woman who had had mastectomies—some reconstructed, some not, some bilateral some not. And not one of them had this skin hanging. All the pictures showed a flat, smooth area with a scar on the chest where a breast used to be.

Mine had fat hanging in various places, skin that looked like an elephant, and hills and valleys that just didn't look like the pictures.

My only comfort is that I truly believe that my David still sees me with breasts. He doesn't see me any other way. He still likes to touch my chest. I hate it. It is just hills and valleys and fat and scars. But he doesn't think that way. It is still an intimate area, and he draws on his memory and feel of physical touch, and he knows that when I do let him touch it, that it is a gift, and he recognizes that.

## August 29

Received a second card on my doorstep. I do not want Kelly back into my life. She is toxic, and I can't have Pastor Sam without her, so I choose to not reestablish those relationships.

*Okay, sometimes people in our life are just toxic. Before this experience, I would never have acted like this. I wouldn't want to hurt their feelings. But here is the thing. Some people are not good for you. And sometimes you need to look out for yourself. It is a healthy thing for you to do to remove them from your life. Pray about it. I recommend a book written by Dr. Henry Cloud and Dr. John Townsend called Boundaries: When to Say Yes, How to Say No, To Take Control of Your Life.*

## September 29

I made an appointment with Mary Ellen at the fitting room. She fitted me for my prosthesis. I remember standing there and she said for me to take off my top. I was hesitant because no one except family and doctors had seen me. I said, "It looks really bad," and she said, "I have seen worse." That was even before she saw me.

She was able to fit me with a special kind of prosthesis that had a pocket in the back so I could put fiberfill in it to even out where the skin was lumpy. It helped, but I never felt so fake in my life. The real me didn't look so good. At the end of my appointment, I asked Mary Ellen if in fact she had seen worse, now that she had seen me. She just gave me a hug and didn't answer.

## October 7

Julie had come over to my house for a visit, and I was particularly down about my chest. She kind of chewed on me because I still had my life. I asked her if she would like to see. And she surprised me by saying yes. So I showed her. She said, "Wow, that is gross." That really meant a lot to me since she had had a mastectomy herself.

## October 12

I decided to find a counselor. And God provided Dr. Wakefield for me to talk to.

## October 17

My first appointment with Dr. Wakefield. He is a great listener. He let me cry when no one else would. He challenged me when I needed it. He gave me homework: to write a letter to either my ex-boss who was abusive or to my breasts. He just wanted me to express my feelings instead of keeping them bottled up. I needed to give words, thoughts, and expressions to my inner thoughts.

*My friend, find a way to express what you are feeling. You can journal, write a letter to God or a friend, or even talk to an empty chair, but it is so important to express them. What about therapy through art? Be creative.*

## October 24

I put off writing my letter until the day of my next session. So at work, I sat and wrote it at lunch. It just poured out of me.

Breasts,

I am really sorry that I chose to have you cut off and incinerated. I failed to be strong. I can't ever go back and undo what I have done. Please forgive me. If it gives you any comfort, I am suffering the consequences for my actions. If God is merciful, He will relieve this pain soon. I didn't really understand that I was killing a part of me. Ignorance is not an excuse, but I truly didn't understand I was breaking who Beth was.

We talked a lot about my letter. He wanted to know what I meant by "breaking who Beth was." I don't know, but

I wasn't me anymore. I had lost my identity. I refer to myself as broken.

Dr. Wakefield gave me another assignment: make a list of everything I lost (by having the mastectomy).

## November 7

David and I worked on the list together.

- Breasts
- Feeling feminine
- Feeling like a woman
- Ability to concentrate
- Loss of joy and contentment
- Loss of intimacy to a degree
- Loss of libido
- Jump-starter gone (My breasts had always been an area that took the lead in my sexual fulfillment.)
- Loss of friends
- Loss of energy
- Can't wear pretty bras (The mastectomy bras come in white or beige.)
- Lingerie doesn't fit the same
- Feeling sexy for David
- Loss of my ability to tease David (My counselor laughed at this one. He said he never heard a woman admit that before.)
- Loss of the feeling of comfort when David reached around me and cupped my breasts
- Decreased health

- My girls are at higher risk (my daughters)
- I now have a secret (Every time a stranger looks at me, I think, *Oh no, they know.*)
- I am fake
- Loss of cleavage (When I bend over, I have a gaping hole.)
- Loss of self-worth
- Loss of a church and church family
- Loss of being pain-free
- Loss of being alive (Now I am part of the walking dead.)
- I can't use the drive-thru at the bank (My incisions have adhered to the chest wall and scar tissue has developed, so I can no longer reach out the left side of the car).
- Can't lift my left arm
- Security
- I betrayed my convictions
- I gave into peer pressure
- Loss of faith at times
- Loss of never having cancer
- Now have a threat that the cancer could return
- Loss of cancer policy
- Loss of my booby bank (David liked to deposit his check down the front of my shirt.)

Dr. Wakefield gave me permission to grieve. I was unaware that I needed permission, but I did. I really did. I wasn't aware of all that I had lost. I wasn't aware of how much pain I was carrying around. My way of dealing was through denial, but that was hard to maintain when the truth was looking at me in the mirror every morning.

*I give you permission to grieve also. Some people will say, "It is no big deal." Some will say, "They just get in the way. You don't need them anymore." But that is just not true. My breasts are important to me. They are part of my body. And like it or not, they in some way define my impression of myself. They do not define who I am, but they do define my impression of who I am. Body image has played a major role in my development as a woman. I would guess that is true for you also. Breasts are important, and they are a big deal!*

## November 14

I keep hearing about finding my new normal. I don't even remember what my old normal was. So Dr. Wakefield and I discussed this. He said to picture a bridge. On one side was what was normal, and on the other side is what will be normal for me after the grieving process. The bridge is the grieving process.

The grieving process is different for everyone, depending on how important the item was that was lost, and one's ability to move on. The only way through grief is through it. Journal my emotions. Be human. Be Beth. It's okay to cry. Forgive myself for the mastectomy. And if David won't let me do this because it is too hard for him, just tell him to get in the boat and be quiet. Tell him that this is what I need. I need him to listen and keep his mouth shut. I need him to be present and not try to fix it. I need my husband. I need support, and I need to grieve.

I know when the blanket of darkness is not over me, that I have made the right decision.

Dr. Wakefield and I talked about getting plastic surgery to remove the excess skin and to get some relief from the pain from scar tissue. I really didn't have a good reason why I hadn't done it before now. I think I was too busy feeling sorry for myself to be able to make that decision. Or maybe it is just hard to do something positive when you feel so negative.

## November 15

Called Dr. Gareth, a reputable plastic surgeon, and made an appointment.

I assigned myself some homework. I decided to make a list that would help me with my bridge to my new normal.

To feel more feminine, I would color my hair, get a manicure, maybe some new clothes that fit right, and get my ears pierced. I got my ears pierced when I was sixteen, but after a year, I couldn't get them to heal so I just let them close up. Thirty years later, I am ready to try again.

Since mastectomy bras are ugly, I think I will buy some pretty regular bras and sew a place into them to hold the prosthesis.

I will find other ways to tease David. Joking, winking, smiling, and touching can all be used to tease. I will learn how to flirt again. Maybe I will buy a feather.

Figure out how to jump-start my motor. Read a book about reviving my libido. Make an active decision to be part of this sexual team.

Stop calling myself a eunuch. Dr. Wakefield suggested wearing a rubber band and snapping it every time a negative thought came to mind. *Eunuch* is snap worthy.

Journal. Maybe I will write a book.

Face the lies I believe about myself, about my self-worth, and about being fake.

## November 18

Saw Dr. Gareth today. He feels confident that he can help relieve the pain and also clean up the area so it won't bother me.

## November 28

Pre-op scheduled. Surgery is scheduled for December 6.

## November 30

My iron was too low for surgery, which would have to be rescheduled. I went to my naturopath, and he recommended an iron supplement from the Cancer Treatment Center that is easier for a body to assimilate. I was now on a mission. I was going to have that surgery. I was going to feel better about myself.

## December 14

Took another blood test to check my iron levels. It has been two weeks of taking iron twice a day, and my iron levels have dropped. The iron levels are so low that my naturopath told me I should not be driving because I could pass out.

I wanted to have the surgery before year-end because I have already met my deductible. Now there is no way. I am so frustrated. I finally had a plan, and yet I seem to run into roadblock after roadblock. More pain, more loss, more frustration. When does this ever stop?

## December 25

No energy, fatigued, depressed. Merry Christmas.

## January-February-March

Another three months have passed, and I have tried everything I could find to get my iron up. Even though it is improved, it is still not high enough for surgery.

## April 4

I have decided to be content. I give up my quest for surgery, and I will live with how I look. I will live with the limited mobility, and I will live with the pain. It is a decision that I have made, and I will keep at it until my emotions follow suit.

I called Mom and Dad and told them about my decision. During our conversation, Dad told me that he wears the vest I gave him often and uses it as a testimony for the Lord. Dad was telling me to read between the lines.

## April 6

Pastor Bob preached a powerful sermon on letting God be in control. I realized that for the last few months, I have been trying to control the surgery. I had forgotten to ask God. When facing a life-threatening illness, it is very difficult to be in control or feel in control, so I did many things to compensate.

## April 7

The nurse from Dr. Gareth's office called. Dr. Gareth had a cancellation and wanted to know how my iron was. I didn't really know, so I went and had my blood tested. I really had mixed emotions about going because I had committed to giving up trying, and yet first chance I got, I jumped at getting another blood test.

## April 8

My iron is perfect. I believe God was waiting to give me the desires of my heart until I stopped and included Him in my desires. I suffer because I don't stop and ask God first.

# April 19

The day I have been waiting for.

When I woke up from surgery, I felt like a weight was lifted off my chest, and I could finally breathe again. Finally! No more pain. No more extra skin or fat. "Why, oh Lord, am I so stubborn? I pray that this time I will have finally learned my lesson."

One year and two days later, and I have learned so much from this journey. My relationship with God is stronger.

*I talked a little bit about the sermon I heard about "writing your life story." Well, I remember another sermon, or rather sermon series, that I heard Pastor Bob preach not long after my cancer journey. It was about "living your life if you only had thirty days to live." He encouraged me to live passionately and love completely. The greatest commandment is found in Mark 12:30, 31, which says, "Love the Lord your God with all your heart and with all your soul and with all your mind and with all your strength . . . and love your neighbor as yourself." That is a tall order.*

*I have found healing in writing this letter. Let me encourage you, my friend, to find what you are passionate about and pursue it. Don't let cancer defeat you. Remember Christ is the big "C." You have the strength of Almighty God at your disposal, if you are in Christ Jesus. I have learned to fill my life passionately and love completely.*

*So, my friend, you have read my challenges, felt my emotions, and heard my heart. I pray you have been encouraged by what I have shared.*

*Dear God,*

*I pray for my friend who has shared this journey with me. Please help her avoid all the mistakes I made. Guide her to doctors with skilled hands and brilliant minds. Help each treatment or surgery to be effective and healing. Give her a clear path to recovery. I pray You will put people in her path that will give her support, encouragement, and friendship. And most of all, Lord, I pray that You will be with her in every moment. Cancer is so lonely. Please pour out your love and blessings on her. Help her to fill her life with passion and love for You. And I pray that she will soon be cancer-free. Please give her life and joy. In Jesus' name.*

*I love you, my friend,*
*Beth*

*Dear Friend,*

*My husband has written me love notes all of our marriage. I asked if he would like to add some comments to this letter, and he decided it was a good opportunity to write another LN. He didn't learn all these points necessarily while we were going through cancer, but he has learned more and more as time goes on.*

*Beth*

*Dear Caregiver and Friend,*

*1. Realize that your love for her is a decision, not just a feeling.*

*This is just one more hurdle to cross in our life together. If my love for her is anything like my Savior's love for me, it is a love regardless. I had made a commitment: "For better or for worse, until death do us part." And this hasn't changed anything.*

*At times such as this, more than ever, she needs my support, understanding, encouragement, and patience. Especially now, she needs to know that I desire her and want her. Her breasts are just a small part of the package.*

*2. Show her that she is not alone in this fight.*

*It is important to show her that this cancer is something that she and I are dealing with together. I will not let it come between us. If she doesn't have to deal with the uncertainty of where her husband is, she will have more energy to deal with the diagnosis, tests, surgeries, and more. I must make sure she understands that this is our problem. I have cancer too. We face all things together.*

*3. Do more than try to fix it.*

*We husbands tend to think that if it is broke, we can fix it. Every problem is solvable. That is why there is duct tape. I have an answer if she will just do what I say.*

*I began to realize that what she most needs from me is a listening ear. If Beth can talk it out (without my interrupting), she can get a handle on it. The key is discussion, not assumption. Probe her real feelings. She need not hide anything from me. No fears, worries, longings, or feelings are sacred. I am there so she has someone to share with.*

*Cancer made her feel fragile and vulnerable. My quiet support helps her cope with these feelings. She needs me for so much more than just help with decisions. I am learning to swallow my advice, cancel my creative alternative, and just hold her, let her cry it out, look her in the eye when she talks, and pray silently as she shares.*

## 4. Reflect her emotional state.

*When surgery went well, we celebrated. When we got bad news, we cried together. Sometimes, I could not cheer her up, so I learned to just be blue with her. At times when I tried to encourage her with Bible verses, she felt preached at. There are times that she needs to process the bad news and work it out in her mind. I am trying to learn her moods, hear her heart, respect her current step progress, always tell her that she is beautiful, and sense where she is.*

## 5. Do not limit your support.

*Be there always. Don't be more supportive before the surgery than afterward. After she is home and healed, when the doctors have done all that they can do, when friends stop coming, still be there for her.*

*It is easy for me to think that since I have helped her prepare and deal with the knife, now that she is home I can go fishing. She is well now. I must understand that although the crisis may have passed and the scars are fading, she still strongly needs me to be there. The issues have just changed color. She still has to deal with feeling ugly, vulnerable, and frustrated. That's where I come in.*

## 6. *Know the Master Controller.*

*I am still learning to cast my cares upon my Lord. In faith, I give my wife's health and future to God. He can deal with it better than I can. I submit to His authority over me and what I want. He had one son without sin, but He has never had a son without sorrow. I am in good company.*

*Some things I just don't know the answer to. Sometimes, I just don't know which way to turn. At times, medical advice is just not any good. But I know that the Creator of the universe is big enough and wise enough to handle me, my wife, our cancer, and all of it.*

*I accept that God knows and understands, and as we yield to Him, His perfect will will be worked out.*

*I have a personal relationship with the Lord Jesus, and that is carrying me through. Our marriage is ordained by Him; we walk close to Him; He is in control. I can be there for Beth, because I know that God is always there for me.*

*Sincerely,*
*David*

*Dear Friend,*

*I can't let my husband have the last word. ☺ I like how he did a one, two, three of what he has learned. So I want to do that also.*

*1. This emotional roller coaster ride will eventually end.*

*Your life will have changed. Your body will be different. But in time, the emotions will even out and your routine will be redefined.*

*2. Sometimes, God calms the storm, sometimes He lets the storm rage, and He calms the child.*

*God is always in control. He knew I would have a lumpectomy, another lumpectomy, a bilateral mastectomy, and another surgery to repair the mastectomy. He knew some of my friends and also the church I had been attending would abandon me. He knew, and He let it happen, and He provided a new church and a conviction in me to help others with cancer.*

*My dad's favorite verse is Romans 8:28. "We know that in all things God works for the good of those who love him, who have been called according to his purpose."*

*3. Working does not equal life.*

*I don't know what has taken over your life that is unhealthy, but I would guess there is something you could do to improve your quality of life. You have been given an opportunity to make changes. Embrace it.*

*4. Develop deep relationships.*

*Invest time in other people's lives. Talk to them often. Friendship is a two-way street. It occurs to me that maybe I didn't have anyone stand by me because I have never stood by anyone.*

*5. Find your purpose for living and do it passionately.*

*If money wasn't an option, what would you do? It might take a lifetime to figure this out. I haven't been able to find my purpose yet, or maybe it changes over time. I don't know but keep looking.*

*My friend, at the beginning of this letter I gave you two promises: to offer you hope and to offer you help. I pray I have fulfilled that promise, help through sharing my journal and this letter and hope by pointing you toward Christ. I found during my time of deepest feelings of abandonment that I still had God. God and God alone will never leave us or forsake us. For God is our hope and our help.*

*Love you My Friend,*
*Beth*

www.ingramcontent.com/pod-product-compliance
Lightning Source LLC
Chambersburg PA
CBHW020350290526
45785CB00005B/2212